ADULT LIMB FRACTURES

D0620592

ADULT LIMB FRACTURES

Ahmed Mujtaba Siddiqui MB BS, FRCS(Ed)
Registrar in Trauma and Orthopaedics
Letterkenny General Hospital, Ireland

Neil Rushton MD, FRCS
Consultant Orthopaedic Surgeon
Orthopaedic Research Unit
Addenbrooke's Hospital
Cambridge

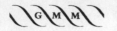

© 2002

Greenwich Medical Media Limited
137 Euston Road
London
NW1 2AA

870 Market Street Ste720
San Francisco
CA 94109, USA

ISBN 1-84110-078-1

First published 2002

The publisher makes no representation, express or implied, with
regard to the accuracy of the information contained in this book and
cannot accept any legal responsibility or liability for any errors or
omissions that may be made.

A catalogue record for this book is available from the British Library.

www.greenwich-medical.co.uk

Distributed Worldwide by Plymbridge Distributors Ltd
and in the USA by Jamco Distribution
Typeset by Phoenix Photosetting, Chatham, Kent
Printed and bound in Great Britain by
The Cromwell Press, Trowbridge, Wiltshire

Contents

UPPER LIMB

Preface

"A classification is useful only if it considers the severity of bone lesion and serves as a basis for treatment and for evaluation of result."

(Maurice. E. Muller)

The classification of fractures has recently been the subject of discussion: which system to use and which not to use. Of the classification systems in use at the moment: the AO system is indeed systematic and comprehensive; it also deals with the different levels and complexities of fractures. It does not, however, deal with pure dislocations or fractures of the scapula, hand or foot. Some malleolar fractures are difficult to categorize and proximal humeral fractures are still a problem. It is also a challenging task for an orthopaedic trainee to grasp this classification.

An ideal classification system should be easily remembered and applied. It should give an insight into the severity of the injury and its prognosis and could be a combination of a number of classification systems.

This book has been written with the object of presenting all the major classifications of fractures of the extremities in one place. It is intended for the orthopaedic surgeon in training to use as a handbook for quick referral. It should also prove to be a revision aid for use prior to orthopaedic board examination, as well as being a valuable reference for all healthcare professionals with a need to understand and interpret different types of limb fractures.

Ahmed M. Siddiqui FRCS (Ed)
Neil Rushton MD, FRCS

Acknowledgements

I express my gratitude to Mr Neil Rushton for his advice and expertise during the production of this book. I am deeply indebted to my teachers: Mr A. Bedford, Mr A. August, Mr S. Sjolin (West Suffolk Hospital), Mr A. McGuinness, Mr J. Curtin (Cork University Hospital), Mr T. Burke (Croom Orthopedic Hospital), Mr J. B. Healy, Mr A. Macey (Sligo General Hospital), Mr J. Buisson, Mr A. Ogden, Mr C. Dreghorn, Mr A. Ratnam (Dumfries and Galloway Royal Infirmary), and many others who taught me the basis of orthopaedics and the value of knowledge. I would also like to thank my family for all their support during this project. My sincere thanks go to the publishers, Greenwich Medical Media Limited.

Ahmed M. Siddiqui, FRCS(Ed)

Lower limb

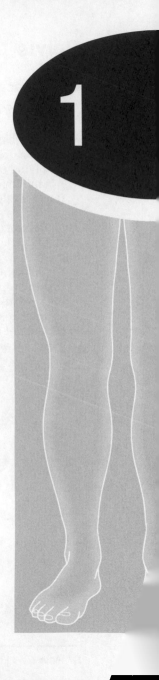

1

Pelvis

Pelvic fractures

Tile's classification

Type A: stable fracture
- A1: fracture of pelvis not involving pelvic ring.
- A2: minimally displaced fracture of pelvic ring.

Type B: rotationally unstable/vertically stable fracture
- B1: AP compression fracture (open book).
- B2: Lateral compression injuries (ipsilateral).
- B3: Lateral compression injuries (contralateral).

Type C: rotationally/vertically unstable fracture
- C1: Unilateral.
- C2: Bilateral.
- C3: Associated with acetabular fracture.

Reference
Tile M. Pelvic ring fractures: should they be fixed? *J Bone Joint Surg* 1988; **70B:** 1–12.

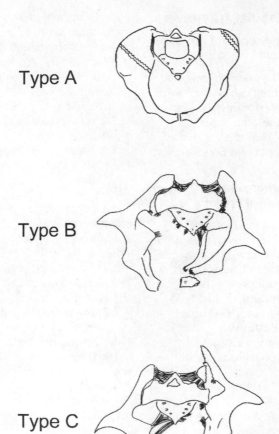

Type A

Type B

Type C

Fig. 1 Tile's classification

Acetabular fractures

Anterior column (iliopubic column)

This is a mass of bone stretching downward from the anterior inferior iliac spine, and includes the pubis and anterior part of the acetabular floor.

Posterior column (ilioischial column)

This is a mass of bone stretching upward from the ischial tuberosity to the sciatic notch, including the posterior part of the acetabulum.

Two commonly used classifications:
1. AO classification.
2. Letournel's classification.

AO classification

Type A: one column is involved
- A1: fracture of posterior wall and certain variations.
- A2: fracture of posterior column and variation.
- A3: fracture of anterior column and variation.

Type B: main fracture line is transverse, acetabular roof always in contact with ilium
- B1: transverse fracture with or without posterior acetabular wall involvement.
- B2: transverse fracture with variation.
- B3: transverse fracture involving anterior column.

Type C: both columns are involved, no part of acetabulum is in contact with the ilium
- C1: fracture involving the anterior column extends to the iliac crest.
- C2: fracture involving the anterior column extends to the anterior border of the ilium.
- C3: fracture involving the sacroiliac joint.

Reference
Muller ME, Allgower M, Schiender R, Willeneger H. *AO Manual of Internal Fixation*, 3rd edn. Berlin, Springer Verlag, 1990.

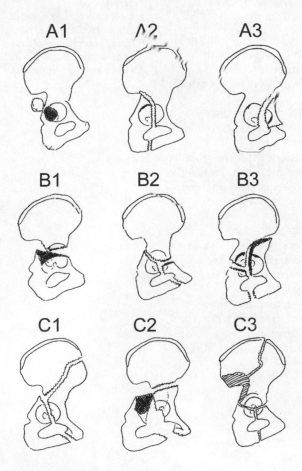

Fig. 2 AO classification

Letournel and Judet classification

- Ten types of fracture.
- Five elementary or simple fractures.
- Five complex fractures.

Elementary fracture
1. Posterior column fracture.
2. Anterior column fracture.
3. Anterior wall fracture.
4. Posterior wall fracture.
5. Transverse fracture.

Complex fracture
1. Posterior column and posterior wall fracture.
2. Transverse and posterior wall fracture.
3. T-shaped fracture.
4. Anterior/posterior hemitransverse fracture.
5. Both column fractures.

Reference
Judet R, Judet J, Letournel E. Fractures of the acetabulum: classification and surgical approaches for open reduction. *J Bone Joint Surg* 1964; **46A:** 1615–1647.

Elementary   Complex

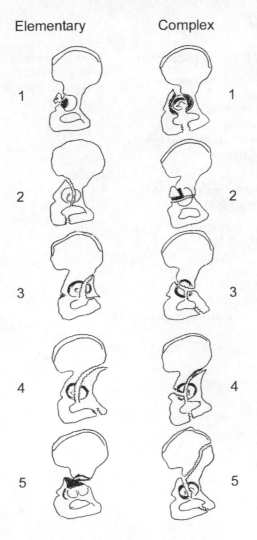

Fig. 3 Letournel and Judet classification

Hip

Fracture dislocations

- Anterior dislocation + fracture.
- Central dislocation + fracture.
- Posterior dislocation + fracture.

Anterior fracture dislocation

Type I: superior dislocation of femoral head
- IA: No associated fracture.
- IB: Femoral head fracture.
- IC: Acetabular fracture.

Type II: inferior dislocation of femoral head
- IIA: No associated fracture.
- IIB: Femoral head fracture.
- IIC: Acetabular fracture.

Reference

Rockwood CA, Green DP. *Fractures in Adults*, 2nd edition, pp 1288–1292.

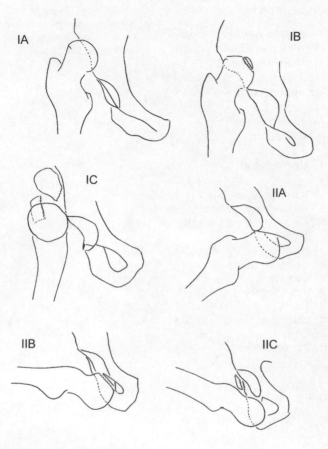

Fig. 4 Anterior fracture dislocation

Central fracture dislocation

A central dislocation is in fact a medial displacement of the femoral head secondary to a displaced acetabular fracture.

Rowe and Lowell classification

1. Undisplaced

2. Inner wall
A: Femoral head beneath dome.
B: Femoral head not beneath dome.

3. Superior dome
A: Congruent.
B: Incongruent.

4. Bursting
A: Congruent.
B: Incongruent.

Reference
Connolly JF (ed) *Depalma's Management of Fractures and Dislocations: An Atlas*, 3rd edition, pp 1348, 1349.

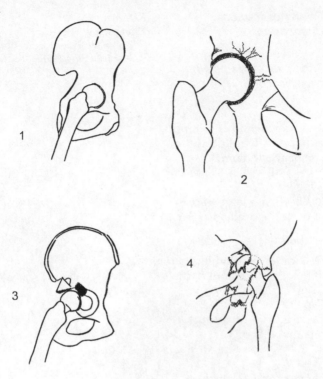

Fig. 5 Rowe and Lowell classification

Posterior fracture dislocation

Thompson and Epstein classification

Type I
Dislocation with or without minor fracture of posterior rim of acetabulum.

Type II
Dislocation + large fracture of posterior acetabular rim.

Type III
Dislocation + comminution of posterior acetabular rim.

Type IV
Dislocation + fracture of acetabular floor.

Type V
Dislocation + fracture of head of femur.

Reference
Thompson VP, Epstein HC. Traumatic dislocation of hip. *J Bone Joint Surg* 1951; **33A:** 746–778.

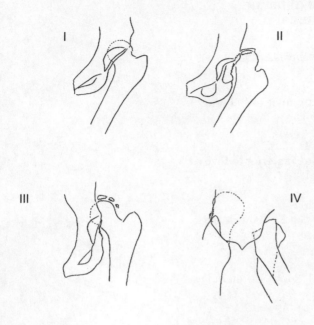

Fig. 6 Thompson and Epstein classification

Head of femur fractures

Pipkin's classification

Type 1
Fracture inferior to fovea centralis.

Type 2
Fracture superior to fovea centralis.

Type 3
Type 1 or 2 + femoral neck fracture.

Type 4
Type 1, 2 or 3 + acetabular fracture.

Reference
Pipkin G. Treatment of grade IV fracture dislocation of hip. *J Bone Joint Surg* 1957; **39:** 1027–1042.

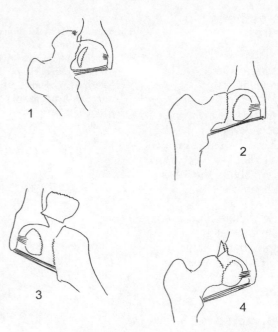

Fig. 7 Pipkin's classification

Periprosthetic hip fractures

Duncan and Masri classification

Type A: fracture involving the trochanter area
- AG: involving the greater trochanter.
- AL: involving the lesser trochanter.

Type B: fracture around or just below the stem
- B1: prosthesis stable.
- B2: prosthesis unstable.
- B3: bone stock inadequate.

Type C: fracture well below the stem

Reference
Duncan CP, Masri BA. Fractures of the femur after hip replacement. In: Jackson DW (ed) *Instructional Course Lectures 44*. Rosemont, IL, American Academy of Orthopedic Surgeons, 1995, pp 293–304.

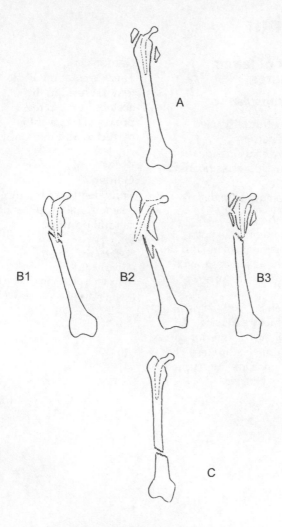

Fig. 8 Duncan and Masri classification

Femur

Neck of femur fractures

Intracapsular

Two commonly used classifications:
1. Garden's classification.
2. Pauwel's classification.

Garden's classification

Garden 1
Inferior cortex is not completely broken, but the trabeculae are angulated (abduction fracture).

Garden 2
The fracture line is complete, the inferior cortex is completely broken. The trabeculae are interrupted but not broken.

Garden 3
There is rotation of the femoral head in the acetabulum; i.e. the proximal fragment is abducted and internally rotated.

Garden 4
Fully displaced fracture. The femoral head lies in a neutral position.

Reference
Garden RS. Reduction and fixation of subcapital fractures of the femur. *Orthop Clin North Am* 1974; **5:** 683–712.

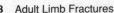

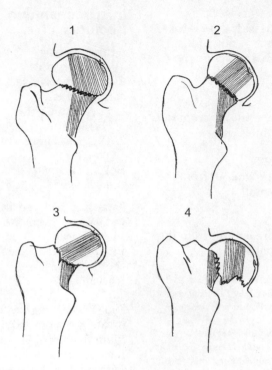

Fig. 9 Garden's classification

Pauwel's classification

This classification is based on the direction of the fracture line across the femoral neck.

Type 1
Fracture line 30° from the horizontal.

Type 2
Fracture line 50° from the horizontal.

Type 3
Fracture line 70° from the horizontal.

Reference
Pauwels F. *Der Schenkelhalsbruch, ein mechanisches Problem. Grundlagen des Heilungsvorganges. Prognose und kausale Therapie*. Stuttgart, Beilageheft zur Zeitschrift für Orthopaedische Chirurgie, Ferdinand Enke, 1935.

Intertrochanteric fractures

Extracapsular

Two commonly used classifications:
1. Boyd and Griffin classification.
2. Jensen's classification.

Boyd and Griffin classification

Type 1: undisplaced, stable fracture with no comminution
Fracture extends along the intertrochanteric line from the greater to lesser trochanter.

Type 2: stable, displaced minimally comminuted fractures
Main fracture along the intertrochanteric line but with multiple fractures in the cortex.

Type 3: unstable large posteromedial fracture

Type 4: intertrochanteric fracture with subtrochanteric extension
NB: Types 3/4 have subtrochanteric extensions.

Reference
Boyd HB, Griffin LL. Classification and treatment of trochanteric fractures. *Arch Surg* 1949; **58**: 853–866.

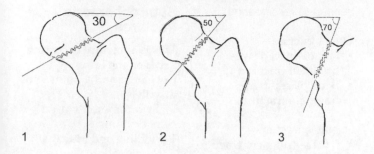

Fig. 10 Pauwel's classification

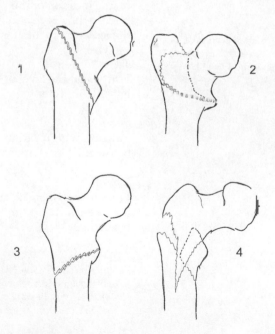

Fig. 11 Boyd and Griffin classification

Jensen's classification

Stable fracture
- I: undisplaced two-fragment fracture.
- II: displaced two-fragment fracture.

Unstable fracture
- I: three-fragment fracture without posterolateral support.
- II: three-fragment fracture without medial support.
- III: four-fragment fracture.

Reference

Jensen JS. Classification of trochanteric fractures. *Acta Orthop Scand* 1980; **51:** 803–810.

Subtrochanteric fractures

This is a fracture occurring between the lesser trochanter and a point 5 cm distally.

Two commonly used classifications:
1. Fielding and Magaliato classification.
2. Seinsheimer's classification.

Fielding and Magaliato classification
This classification is based on the location of the fracture line in relation to the lesser trochanter.

Type 1
Fracture at the level of the lesser trochanter.

Type 2
Fracture within 2.5 cm below the lesser trochanter.

Type 3
Fracture between 2.5 and 5 cm below the lesser trochanter.

Reference

Fielding JW, Magaliato HJ. Subtrochanteric fractures. *Surg Gynecol Obstet* 1966; **122:** 555–560.

Stable

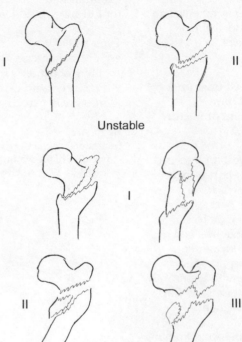

Unstable

Fig. 12 Jensen's classification

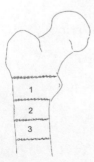

Fig. 13 Fielding and Magaliato classification

Seinsheimer's classification
This classification is based
on fracture fragments and
location and shape of
fracture lines.

Type I
Undisplaced fracture with
less than 2 mm
displacement of fracture
fragments.

Type II: two-part fracture
- IIA: two-part transverse
  femoral fracture.
- IIB: two-part spiral
  fracture with lesser
  trochanter attached to
  proximal fragment.
- IIC: two-part spiral
  fracture with lesser
  trochanter attached to
  distal fragment.

Type III: three-part fracture
- IIIA: three-part spiral
  fracture in which the
  lesser trochanter is part
  of the third fragment,
  which has an inferior
  spike of cortex of varying
  length.
- IIIB: three-part spiral
  fracture in which the
  third part is a butterfly
  fragment.

Type IV
Comminuted fracture with
four or more fragments.

Type V
- Subtrochanteric–
  intertrochanteric fracture.
- Fractures with extension
  into greater trochanter.

Reference
Seinsheimer F. Subtrochanteric
fractures of the femur. *J Bone
Joint Surg* 1978; **60A:** 300–306.

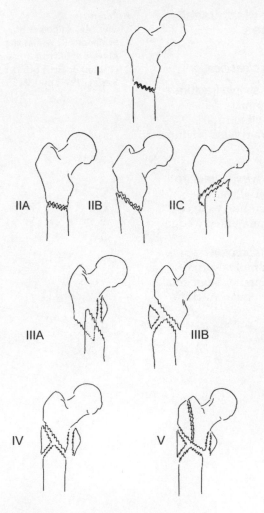

Fig. 14 Seinsheimer's classification

Femur diaphyseal fractures

Muller's classification

Type A: simple fracture
- A1: spiral.
- A2: oblique >30°.
- A3: transverse fracture <30°.

Type B: wedge fracture
- B1: spiral wedge.
- B2: bending wedge.
- B3: fragmented wedge.

Type C: complex fracture
- C1: complex spiral.
- C2: complex segmental.
- C3: irregular fracture.

Reference

Muller ME, Allgower M, Schiender R, Willeneger H. *AO Manual of Internal Fixation*, 3rd edition. Berlin, Springer Verlag, 1991, pp 138–139.

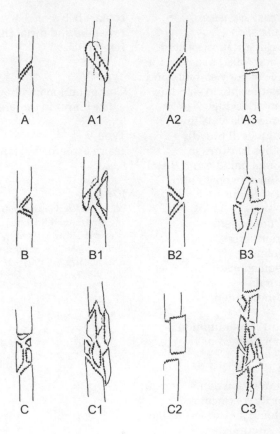

Fig. 15 Muller's classification

Winquist–Hansen classification

This classification system was developed to assess the degree of bony stability and its relationship to standard and interlocking intramedullary nailing techniques. It broadly classifies fractures in proximal, middle and distal one-third, in relation to shaft of femur.

Fracture pattern
- Transverse.
- Oblique.
- Segmental.
- Spiral.
- Comminuted.

Fracture comminution is further defined by degree.

Type I
Comminution denotes small butterfly fragment involving 25% or less of the bony circumference.

Type II
Comminuted fragments involve up to 50% of the width of the bone.

Type III
Comminuted fragment involves more than 50% of the width of the bone that leaves only a small area of contact between the proximal and distal fracture fragments.

Type IV
Comminution involves the entire bony circumference.

Type V
There is segmental bone loss.

Reference
Winquist RA, Hansen St Jr. Comminuted fractures of the femoral shaft treated by intramedullary nailing. *Orthop Clin North Am* 1908; **11:** 633–647.

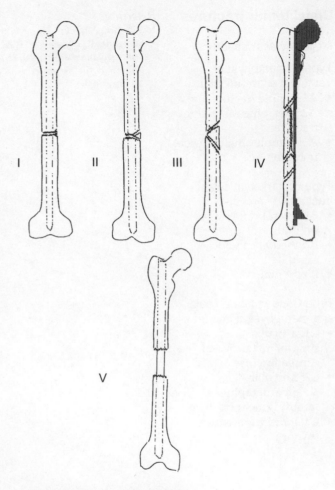

Fig. 16 Winquist–Hansen classification

Distal femur fractures

Muller's classification

Type A: metaphyseal fractures; extra-articular
- A1: simple fracture.
- A2: metaphyseal wedge fracture.
- A3: complex metaphyseal fracture.

Type B: partial articular fractures
- B1: lateral condyle—sagittal.
- B2: medial condyle—sagittal.
- B3: frontal.

Type C: complete articular and metaphyseal fractures
- C1: articular simple/metaphyseal simple fracture.
- C2: articular simple/metaphyseal multifragment fracture.
- C3: multifragmentary fracture.

Reference
Muller ME, Allgower M, Schiender R, Willeneger H. *AO Manual of Internal Fixation*, 3rd edition. Berlin, Springer Verlag, 1990.

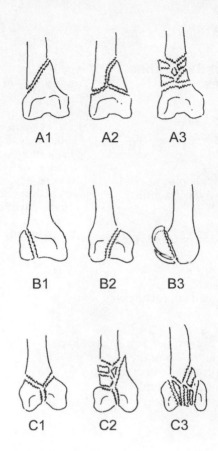

Fig. 17 Muller's classification

Knee

Periprosthetic knee fractures

Neer and Merkel classification

Type I
Minimally displaced supracondylar fracture.

Type II
Displaced supracondylar fracture.

Type III
Comminuted supracondylar fractures.

Type IV
Fracture at the tip of the femoral prosthetic stem or fracture of the femoral diaphysis above the prosthesis.

Type V
Any fracture of the tibia.

References

Merkel KD, Johnson EW. Supracondylar fracture of femur after total knee arthroplasty. *J Bone Joint Surg* 1986; **68A:** 29–43.

Neer C, Granton S, Shelton M. Supracondylar fractures of adult femur. *J Bone Joint Surg* 1967; **49A:** 591.

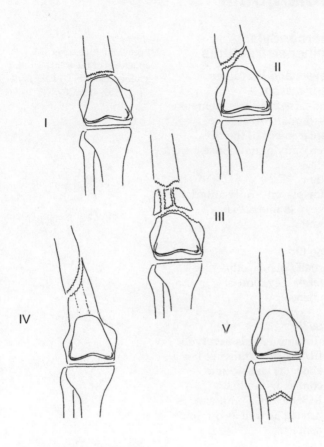

Fig. 18 Neer–Merkel classification

Tibia/fibula

Intercondylar eminence fractures

Meyers and McKeever classification
This classification scheme is based on the degree of displacement of the tibial intercondylar eminence.

Type I
Undisplaced—only anterior edge of eminence is elevated.

Type II
Partially displaced—anterior elevation of eminence.

Type III
Entire eminence is involved.
- IIIA: entire eminence lies above its bed—out of contact with tibia.
- IIIB: the tibial eminence is rotated as well as out of contact.

Reference
Meyers MH, McKeever IM. Fractures of the intercondylar eminence of tibia, *J Bone Joint Surg* 1959; **41A:** 209.

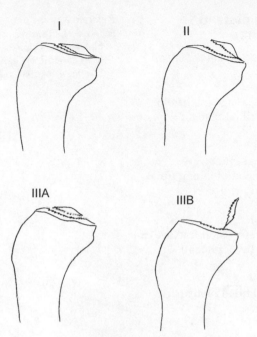

Fig. 19 Meyers–McKeever classification

Tibia/fibula

Tibial plateau fractures

Schatzker's classification

Type I
Pure cleavage fracture of lateral tibial plateau.

Type II
Cleavage fracture + depression of lateral tibial plateau.

Type III
Pure depression fracture of lateral tibial plateau.

Type IV
Medial tibial plateau fracture.

Type V
Bicondylar fracture.

Type VI
Extension of the fracture line to the diaphysis.

Reference
Schatzker J. Fractures of the tibial plateau. In: Schatzker J, Tile M (eds) *Rationale of Operative Fracture Care*. 1987, p 279.

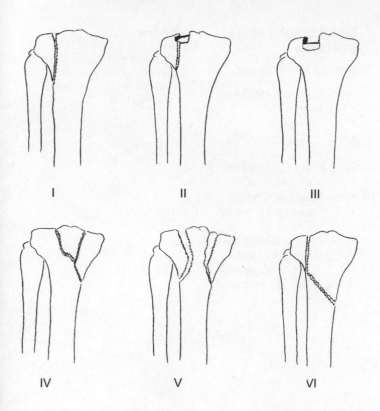

I II III

IV V VI

Fig. 20 Schatzker's classification

Tibial diaphyseal fractures

Muller's classification

Type A: simple fractures
- A1: spiral.
- A2: oblique >30°.
- A3: transverse <30°.

Type B: wedge fracture
- B1: spiral wedge.
- B2: bending wedge.
- B3: fragmented wedge.

Type C: complex fracture
- C1: complex spiral.
- C2: complex segmental.
- C3: irregular fracture.

Reference

Muller ME, Allgower M, Schiender R, Willeneger H. *AO Manual of Internal Fixation*. 3rd edition. Berlin, Springer Verlag, 1990.

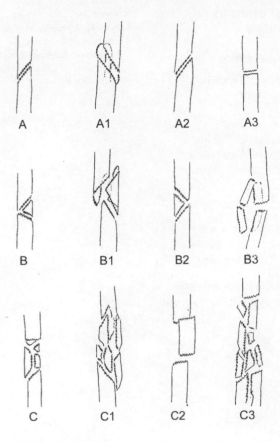

Fig. 21 Muller's classification

Tibial plafond fractures

Pilon fractures

Ruedi and Allgower classification

Type I
Undisplaced T-shaped fracture of distal tibia extending into the joint.

Type II
Same as type I + displacement of intra-articular components.

Type III
Complete intra-articular multifragmentary fracture.

Reference
Ruedi TP, Allgower M. The operative treatment of the intra-articular fractures of the lower end of tibia. *Clin Orthop* 1979; **138:** 105–110.

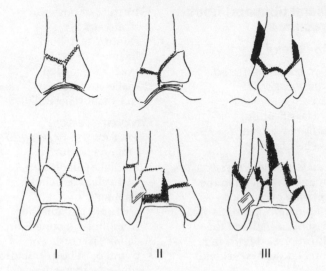

I   II   III

Fig. 22 Ruedi–Allgower classification

Distal tibia and fibula fractures

Ankle joint

Two commonly used classifications:
1. Lauge-Hansen classification.
2. Danis–Weber classification.

Lauge-Hansen classification
In this classification the position of the foot (supination/pronation) is described first and the direction of deforming forces described second.

Supination (inversion)/ adduction injuries (SA)
- Transverse avulsion type fracture of the fibula below the level of the syndesmosis.
- Vertical fracture of the medial malleolus.

Supination (inversion)/ external rotation injuries (SER)
- Disruption of anterior tibiofibular ligament (avulsion of tibial attachment of ligament produces Tillaux fracture).
- Spiral or oblique fracture of distal fibula—fracture line running anteroinferior to posterosuperior.
- Disruption of posterior tibiofibular ligament or fracture of posterior malleolus.
- Rupture of deltoid ligament or avulsion fracture of medial malleolus (the talus is now free to move laterally).

Pronation (eversion)/ external rotation injuries (PER)
- Oblique fracture of medial malleolus or disruption of deltoid ligament.
- Disruption of anterior tibiofibular ligament or Tillaux fracture.
- Spiral or oblique fracture of fibula above the level of syndesmosis—fracture line is anterosuperior to posteroinferior (opposite to SER).
- The fibula may fracture proximally (Maisonneuve fracture).
- Disruption of posterior tibiofibular ligament or fracture of posterior malleolus.
- Disruption of interosseous membrane with gross diastasis (Dupuytren fracture dislocation).

Pronation (eversion)/ abduction injuries (PA)
- Disruption of deltoid ligament or avulsion (transverse) fracture of medial malleolus.

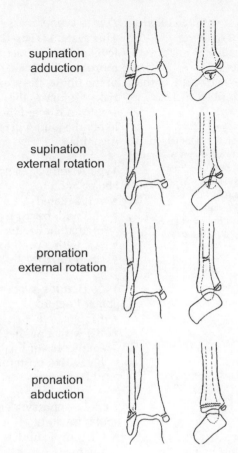

supination
adduction

supination
external rotation

pronation
external rotation

pronation
abduction

Fig. 23 Lauge-Hansen classification

- Rupture of syndesmotic ligament (anterior / posterior tibiofibular ligament).
- Short horizontal or oblique fracture of fibula.

Pronation (eversion)/dorsiflexion injuries (compression) (PD)
- Shearing fracture of medial malleolus.
- Fracture of anterior margin of tibia.
- ? Subluxation of talus

anteriorly with the tibial marginal fracture.
- Supramalleolar fracture of the fibula.
- Transverse fracture of the posterior tibial surface.

References

Lauge-Hansen N. 'Ligamentous' ankle fractures, diagnosis and treatment. *Acta Chir Scand* 1949; **97**: 544–550.

Lauge-Hansen N. Fractures of the ankle: V. Pronation-dorsiflexion fractures. *Arch Surg* 1953; **67**: 813–820.

Danis–Weber classification

This system is based on the level of fibular fracture—the more proximal the fracture of the fibula, the greater the risk of injury to the syndesmosis and the more likely the joint will be unstable.

Type A: infrasyndesmotic fibular fracture
- A1: isolated.
- A2: with fracture of medial malleolus.
- A3: with a posteromedial tibial fracture.

Type B: trans-syndesmotic fibular fracture
- B1: isolated.
- B2: with a medial lesion (malleolus or ligament).
- B3: with a posteromedial tibial fracture.

Type C: suprasyndesmotic fibular fracture
- C1: simple fibular fracture.
- C2: complex fibular fracture.
- C3: proximal fibular fracture.

The Lauge-Hansen accounts for 95% of ankle injuries. However it is a complex classification and not all fractures fit the classical

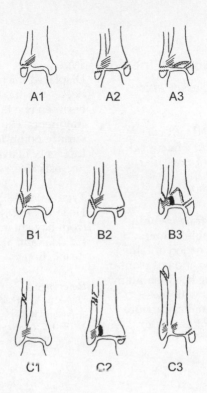

Fig. 24 Danis–Weber classification

patterns. The Danis–Weber system is simpler and is useful in planning surgical treatment.

Type A = SA.
Type B = SER.
Type C = PER.

Reference

Weber BG. *Die Verletzungen des oberen Sprunggellenkes: Aktuelle Probleme in der Chirurgie.* Bern, Verlag Hans Huber, 1966.

Foot

Talus fractures (neck)

Hawkins' classification

Type 1
Undisplaced vertical fracture of the talar neck. Incidence of avascular necrosis 10%.

Type 2
Displaced fracture with subtalar subluxation; proximal portion of talus adopts a position of plantar flexion. The head maintains its position with the navicular and calcaneum. Incidence of avascular necrosis 50%.

Type 3
Displaced fracture of talar neck—the tibia is driven between two talar fragments. The fractured surface points laterally. Incidence of avascular necrosis 85%.

Type 4
Head of talus dislocates from navicular. There is subtalar and ankle joint dislocation.

Reference
Hawkins LG. Fractures of the neck of talus. *J Bone Joint Surg* 1970; **52A:** 991–1002.

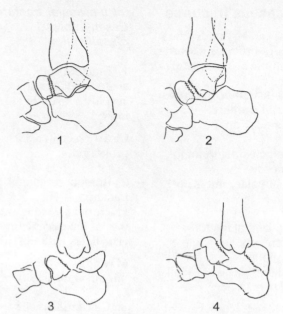

Fig. 25 Hawkins' classification

Foot

Calcaneus fractures

These can be divided into:
- Extra-articular fractures.
- Intra-articular fractures.

Extra-articular fractures: Essex-Lopresti classification

1. Vertical fracture of the tuberosity
The subtalar joint is not involved.

2. Horizontal fracture: posterosuperior angle of calcaneum
No disturbance of Achilles tendon insertion.

Avulsion fracture caused by sudden muscle contraction.

3. Calcaneum body fracture: no involvement of the subtalar joint
Fracture line passes just posterior to the talocalcaneal joint.

Proximal displacement of the calcaneum portion carrying the Achilles tendon.

Intra-articular fractures: Essex-Lopresti classification

1. Fractures of sustentaculum tali
Usually a result of eversion injury.

Clearly seen in axial projection.

2. Anterior calcaneal fractures
Fracture affects the anterior part of the calcaneum which articulates with the cuboid.

May be associated with midtarsal instability.

3. Calcaneal fracture with displacement and subtalar joint involvement
A primary fracture line begins in the sinus tarsi and extends obliquely and posteriorly to exit the medial wall; hence the fracture travels anterolateral to posteromedial.

The calcaneum is separated into two main fragments:

the tuberosity fragment lateral to the centre of talus;

the sustentacular fragment medial to the centre of talus.

A secondary fracture line may also appear; this results

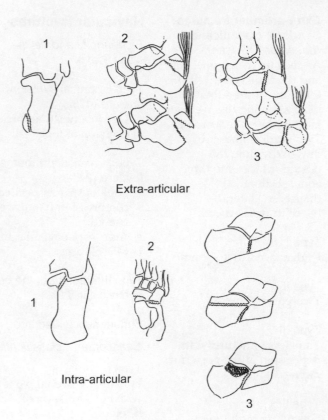

Extra-articular

Intra-articular

Fig. 26 Essex-Lopresti classification

from axial force that is maintained after the primary fracture line occurs. Includes tongue fracture and joint depression fractures.

Reference

Essex-Lopresti P. The mechanism, reduction technique and results in the fractures of the os calcis. *Br J Surg* 1952; **39**: 395–419.

Extra-articular fractures: Sanders' classification

(based on CT scan)

As seen on the coronal (left) and the transverse (right) CT scans of the subtalar joint, showing the posterior facet in the widest profile. Two vertical lines are drawn dividing the posterior facet into three equal sections (hence: A—lateral; B—central; C—medial).

Type I
Undisplaced (not shown).

Type II
Two-part fractures.

Type III
Three-part fractures with depression of the posterior facet.

Type IV
Severely comminuted fractures.

Reference

Sanders R, Fortin P, DiPasquale T, Walling A. Operative treatment in 120 displaced intra-articular calcaneal fractures. *Clin Orthop* 1993; **290:** 87–95.

Navicular fractures

Eichenholtz and Levine classification

Type I: cortical avulsion fracture (47%)
• Due to a twisting force or eversion of foot.

Type II: navicular tuberosity fracture (24%)
• Look out for associated compression fracture of cuboid.
• Accessory navicular in 64% of cases.

Type III: fracture of the body of navicular (29%)

Further subdivided into:

Sangeorzan's classification

Type I
Fracture in coronal plane with no angulation of forefoot.

Type II
Fracture line is dorsolateral to plantaromedial and forefoot is displaced medially.

Type IIIF
Fracture is comminuted and forefoot is displaced laterally.

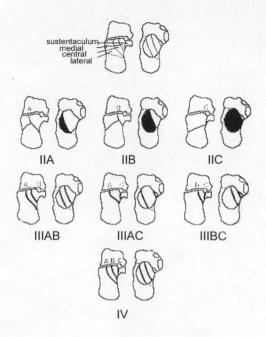

Fig. 27 Sanders' classification

References

Eichenholtz SN, Levine DB. Fractures of tarsal navicular bone. *Clin Orthop* 1964; **34:** 142–157.

Sangeorzan BJ. Displaced intra-articular fractures of the tarsal navicular. *J Bone Joint Surg* 1989; **71A:** 1504–1510.

Foot

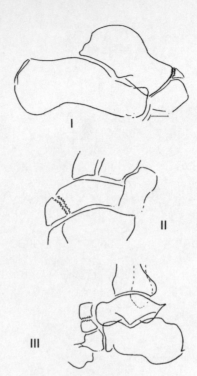

I

II

III

Fig. 28 Eichenholtz–Levine classification

Tarsometatarsal joint injuries

Lisfranc injuries

Quenu and Kuss classification

Type I: homolateral
All five metatarsals displaced in same direction.

Type II: isolated
One or two metatarsals displaced from the others.

Type III: divergent
Displacement of metatarsal in both sagittal/coronal planes.

Reference
Quenu E, Kuss E. Etude sur les luxations du métatarse (luxations métatarso-tarsiennes) du diastasis entre le 1. et le 2. métatarsien. *Rev Chir Paris* 1909; **39:** 281–336, 720–791, 1093–1134.

Foot

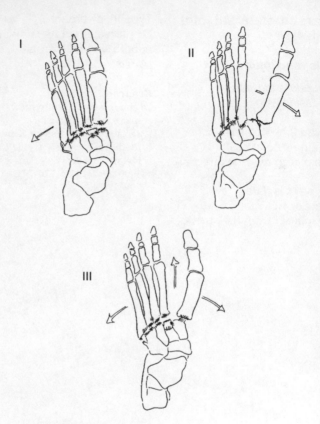

Fig. 29 Quenu–Kuss classification

Proximal fifth metatarsal fractures

Dameron–Lawrence–Botte classification

Zone I: avulsion fractures

Zone II: fracture at the metaphyseal/diaphyseal junction (acute injury)

Zone III: stress fracture of the proximal 1.5 cm of shaft (Jones fracture)

References

Dameron TB Jr. Fractures of the proximal fifth metatarsal: selecting the best treatment options. *J Am Acad Orthop Surg* 1995; **3**: 110–114.

Lawrence ST, Botte MJ. Jones' fractures and related fractures of the proximal fifth metatarsal. *Foot Ankle* 1993; **14**: 358–365.

Foot

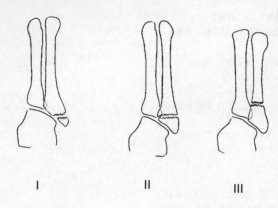

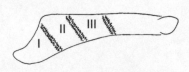

Fig. 30 Dameron–Lawrence–Botte classification

Upper limb

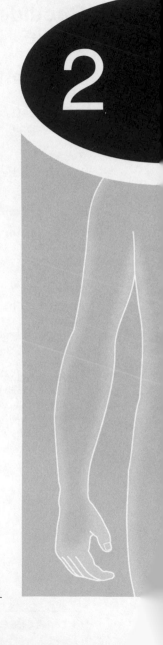

2

Shoulder girdle

Fracture of the scapula

Zdrakovic–Damholt classification

Type I
Fracture of the body
(49–89%).

Type II
Fracture of the apophysis
including the coracoid and
acromion.

Type III
Fracture of the superolateral
angle including the neck
(10–60%)/glenoid.

References
Zdrakovic D, Damholt VV.
    Comminuted and severely
    displaced fractures of the
    scapula. *Acta Orthop Scand*
    1974; **45:** 60–65.

Fracture of glenoid (intra-articular: subdivision of type III fracture of scapula)

Ideberg's classification

Type I
Fracture of glenoid rim:
- IA: anterior.
- IB: posterior.

Type II
Transverse fracture through the glenoid fossa with an inferior triangular fragment displaced with the humeral head.

Type III
Oblique fracture through the glenoid, exiting at the mid-superior border of the scapula; often associated with acromioclavicular fracture or dislocation.

Type IV
Horizontal fracture exiting through the medial border of the scapula.

Type V
Type IV + fracture separating the inferior half of glenoid.

Type VI (Goss)
Severe comminution of glenoid surface.

References

Goss TP. Double disruptions of the superior shoulder suspensory complex. *J Orthop Trauma* 1993; **7**: 99–106.

Ideberg R. Fractures of the scapula involving glenoid fossa. In: Bateman JE, Welsh RP (eds) *Surgery of the Shoulder*. Toronto, BC Decker, 1984, pp 63–66.

Shoulder girdle

Glenoid fractures

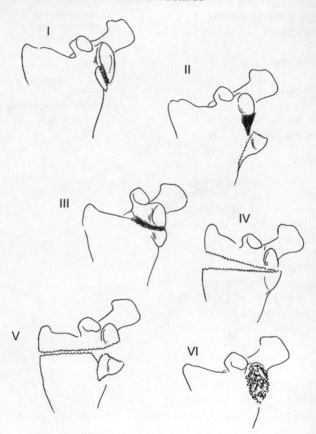

Fig. 31 Ideberg's classification

Clavicular fractures

Allman's classification

Group I: fracture of the middle third (80%)

Group II: fracture of the distal third (12–15%) Subclassified in relation to the location of the coracoclavicular ligament to the fracture fragment.

Neer's classification of the distal third of the clavicle

Type I
Interligamentous fracture occurs between the coracoclavicular and acromioclavicular ligaments. The stable fracture b/c ligament remains attached to the medial fragment.

Type II
Fracture medial to coracoclavicular ligament (unstable).
• IIA: both ligaments (coroid and trapezoid) attached to distal fragment.
• IIB: coroid torn, trapezoid attached to distal fragment.

Type III
Fracture involves the acromioclavicular joint without coracoclavicular ligament injury.

Group III: fracture of proximal third (5–6%)

References
Allman FL. Fractures and ligamentous injuries of the clavicle and its articulation. *J Bone Joint Surg* 1967; **49A:** 774–784.
Neer CS II. Fractures of the distal clavicle with detachment of coracoclavicular ligaments in adults. *J Trauma* 1963; **3:** 99–110.

Shoulder girdle

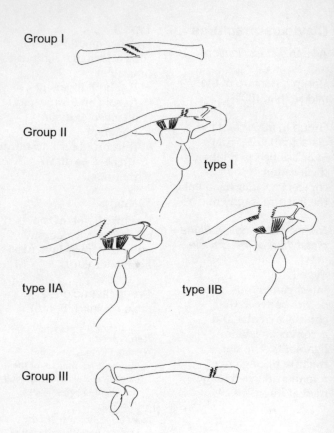

Fig. 32 Allman's classification

Shoulder

Periprosthetic shoulder fractures

Classification (modified from Johansson and colleagues)

Type I
Fracture proximal to the tip of the humeral prosthesis.

Type II
Fracture in the proximal portion of the humerus with distal extension beyond the tip of the prosthesis.

Type III
Fracture occurring entirely distal to the tip of the prosthesis.

Type IV
Fracture occurring adjacent to the glenoid prosthesis.

Reference
Rockwood CA, Green DP.
 Rockwood and Green's Fractures in Adults, 4th edition.
 Philadelphia, JB Lippincott.

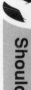

Shoulder

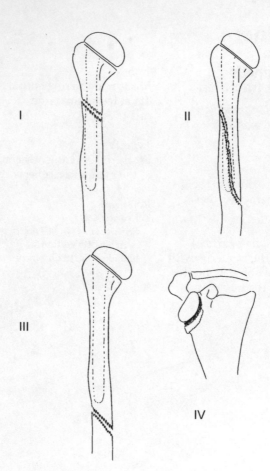

Fig. 33 Periprosthetic shoulder fracture classification

Humerus

Proximal humeral fractures

Neer's classification

Group I
All fractures in this region—with displacement <1 cm and angulation <45°.

Group II
All fractures of anatomical neck—displaced >1 cm.

Group III
All displaced and angulated fractures of surgical neck.

Group IV
All fractures of greater tuberosity, displaced by pull of supraspinatus.

Group V
All fractures involving lesser tuberosity.

Group VI
Fracture dislocation of shoulder.

Reference
Neer CS. Displaced proximal humeral fractures: I. Classification and evaluation. *J Bone Joint Surg* 1970; **52A:** 1077–1089.

Humerus

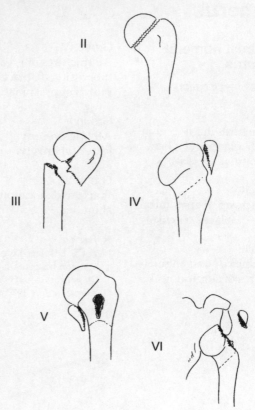

Fig. 34 Neer's classification

Humeral diaphyseal fractures

Muller's classification

Type A: simple (non-comminuted)
- A1: spiral.
- A2: oblique >30°.
- A3: transverse fracture <30°.

Type B: wedge fracture
- B1: spiral wedge.
- B2: bending wedge.
- B3: fragmented wedge.

Type C: complex fracture
- C1: complex spiral.
- C2: complex segmental.
- C3: complex irregular.

Reference
Muller ME, Nazarian S, Koch P, Schatzker J. *The Comprehensive Classification of Fractures of Long Bones*. Berlin, Springer-Verlag, 1990.

Humerus

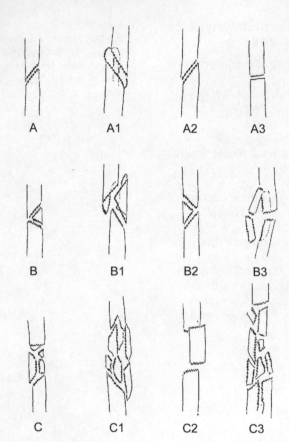

Fig. 33 Muller's classification

Distal humeral fractures

Supracondylar fractures

Fractures occur in the distal humeral metaphysis, above the joint capsule, and are completely extra-articular.

Kocher's classification
Fracture line is transverse and fracture can be displaced or undisplaced.

Type I: extension-type supracondylar fracture (96%)
Distal fragment is displaced posteriorly.

Type II: flexion-type supracondylar fracture (4%)
Distal fragment is displaced anteriorly.

Type III: rotational—with extension or flexion

Reference
Rockwood and Green's Fractures in Adults, 3rd edition. Philadelphia, JB Lippincott, 1991, pp 744–751.

Humerus

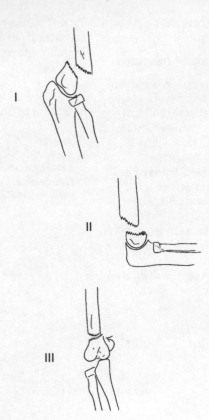

Fig. 34 Kocher's classification

Intercondylar T- or Y-fractures

Riseborough and Radin classification

Type I
Undisplaced fracture between the capitellum and trochlea.

Type II
Separation of the capitellum and trochlea without appreciable rotation of the fragments in the frontal plane.

Type III
Separation of the fragments with rotational deformity.

Type IV
Severe comminution of the articular surface with wide separation of the humeral condyles.

Reference
Riseborough EJ, Radin EL. Intercondylar T fractures of the humerus in the adult: a comparison of operative and non-operative treatment in twenty-nine cases. *J Bone Joint Surg* 1969; **51A:** 130–141.

Humerus

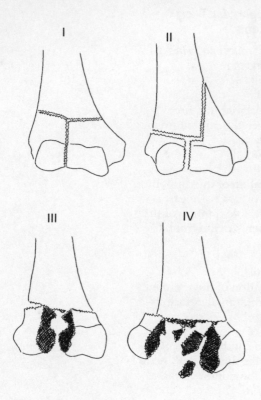

Fig. 35 Riseborough–Radin classification

Humeral condylar fractures

Milch's classification

Lateral condyle

Type I:
Fracture through the capitellum; lateral trochlear ridge remains intact preventing dislocation of the radius and ulna.

Type II:
Simple, transtrochlear—lateral metaphyseal fracture with medial capsuloligamentous disruption of the radius and the ulna dislocates laterally.

Medial condyle

Type I:
Partial fracture of the trochlea; trochlear ridge remains intact to provide medial to lateral stability of the radius and ulna.

Type II:
Simple, transtrochlear—medial metaphyseal fracture with lateral capsuloligamentous disruption of the radius and the ulna dislocates medially.

Reference
Milch H. Fractures and fracture-dislocation of the humeral condyles. *J Trauma* 1964; **4:** 592–607.

Humerus

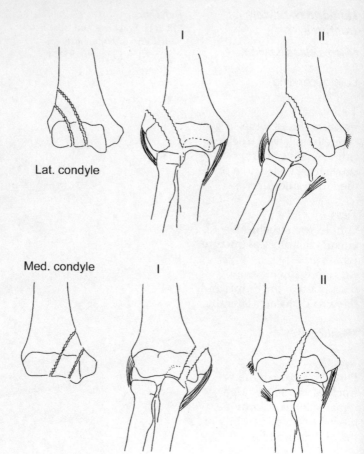

Lat. condyle

I

II

Med. condyle

I

II

Fig. 36 Milch's classification

Fractures of the capitellum

Type I: Hahn–Steinthal fracture
Complete fracture of the capitellum, with extension into the trochlea.

Type II: Kocher–Lorenz fracture
Incomplete fracture of the capitellum in that very little subchondral bone is attached to the capitellar fragment.

The capitellar fragment is usually displaced anteriorly but occasionally the fracture fragment can be displaced posteriorly. In this instance an obstruction to extension is noted on physical examination.

References

Hahn NF. Fall von einer besonderen Varietät der Frakturen des Ellenbogens. *Z Wundarzte Geburtshilfe* 1853; **6:** 185–189.

Kocher T. *Beiträge zur Kenntniss einiger tischwichtiger Frakturforamen*. Basel, Sallman, 1896, pp 585–591.

Lorenz H. Zur Kenntniss der fractura humeri (eminentiae capitata). *Dtsch Z Chir* 1905; **78:** 531–545.

Steinthal D. Die isolierte Fraktur der eminentia capitata im Ellenbogengelenk. *Zentralbl Chir* 1898; **15:** 17–20.

Fractures of the trochlea

Laugier's fracture
- Isolated fractures of the trochlea are very rare.
- Fracture may extend from the trochlea to the distal portion of the epicondyle.
- Displaced fracture lies on the medial side of the joint just distal to the medial epicondyle.

Reference

Stimson LA. *A Treatise on Fractures*. Philadelphia, Henry C Lea, 1890 (Stimson credited the original description to Laugier in 1853).

Humerus

type I

type II

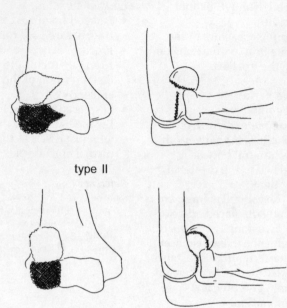

Fig. 37 Capitellum fractures

Elbow

Periprosthetic elbow fractures

Type I
Fracture of the humerus proximal to the humeral component.

Type II
Fracture of the humerus or ulna in any location along the length of the prosthesis (including those fractures that extend proximal or distal to the humeral and ulnar components, respectively).

Type III
Fracture of the ulna distal to the ulnar component.

Type IV
Fracture of the implant.

Reference
Rockwood and Green's Fractures in Adults, 4th edition. Philadelphia, JB Lippincott.

Elbow

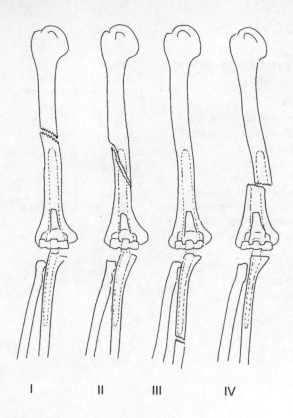

Fig. 38 Periprosthetic elbow fractures

Radius and ulna

Olecranon fractures

Colton's classification

Type I: undisplaced/stable
Involves proximal third of
the articular surface.

Type II: displaced
Involves middle third:
- IIA: fracture is displaced
  but no depression.
- IIB: depression.

Type III: fracture involving
distal third

*Hume fracture dislocation.
Fracture of the olecranon with
anterior dislocation of the
radial head.*

Reference
Colton CL. Fractures of the
  olecranon in adults:
  classification and
  management. *Injury* 1973; **5:**
  121–129.

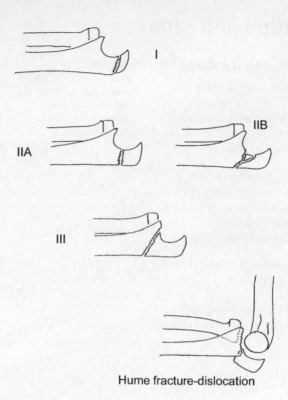

Hume fracture-dislocation

Fig. 39 Colton's classification

Coronoid fractures

Regan and Morrey classification

Type I
Simple avulsion fracture of the coronoid.

Type II
Fracture involving half or less of the coronoid.

Type III
Fracture involving more than half of the coronoid.

Reference
Regan W, Morrey BF. Fractures of the coronoid process of the ulna. *J Bone Joint Surg* 1989; **71A:** 1348.

Radial head fractures

Mason's classification

Type I
Hairline fracture.

Type II
Marginal radial head fracture with minimal displacement, depression or angulation.

Type III
Comminuted radial head fracture.

Type IV
Radial head fracture with elbow dislocation.

Comminuted fractures of radial head are usually associated with the Essex-Lopresti lesion:

- Comminuted fracture of the radial head.
- Disruption of the interosseous membrane.
- Disruption of the distal radio-ulnar joint.
- Proximal translation of the radius.

Reference
Mason ML. Some observations on fractures of the head of the radius with a review of one hundred cases. *Br J Surg* 1954; **42:** 123–132.

Radius and ulna

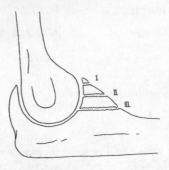

Fig. 40 Regan–Morrey classification

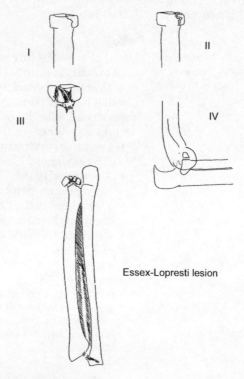

Essex-Lopresti lesion

Fig. 41 Mason's classification

Radius/ulna fracture dislocation

Monteggia fractures (1814)

Fracture of the proximal third of the ulna with anterior dislocation of the radial head.

Bado's classification

Type I
Fracture of the ulnar diaphysis at any level with anterior angulation at the fracture site with associated anterior dislocation of the radial head.

Type II
Fracture of the ulnar diaphysis with posterior angulation at the fracture site and posterolateral dislocation of the radial head.

Type III
Fracture of the ulnar metaphysis with lateral or anterolateral dislocation of the radial head.

Type IV
Fracture of the proximal third of the radius and ulna at the same level with an anterior dislocation of the radial head.

Reference
Bado JL. The Monteggia lesion. *Clin Orthop* 1967; **50**: 71–86.

Radius and u....

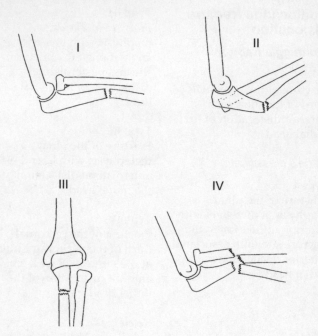

Fig. 42 Bado's classification

Galeazzi's fracture (1934)

Solitary fracture of the radius at the junction of the middle and distal thirds with dislocation of the distal radioulnar joint.

Reference

Galeazzi R. Über ein besonderes Syndrom bei Verletzungen im Bereich der Unterarmknochen. *Arch Orthop Unfallchir* 1934; **35:** 557–562.

Diaphyseal fractures of the radius/ulna

Muller's classification

Type A
Simple fracture involving one or both bones.
- A1: simple fracture of the ulna with intact radius.
- A2: simple fracture of the radius with ulna intact.
- A3: simple fracture of both bones.

Type B
Wedge fractures; one or both bones involved.
- B1: wedge fracture of the ulna; intact radius.
- B2: wedge fracture of the radius; intact ulna.
- B3: wedge fracture of one bone with simple or wedge fracture of the other.

Type C
Complex fractures.
- C1: complex fracture of the ulna.
- C2: complex fracture of the radius.
- C3: complex fracture of both bones.

Reference

Muller ME, Allgower M, Schiender R, Willeneger H. *AO Manual of Internal Fixation*, 3rd edition. Berlin, Springer Verlag, 1990.

Radius and ulna

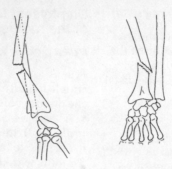

Fig. 43 Galeazzi's fracture

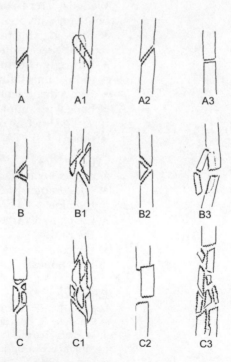

Fig. 44 Muller's classification

Distal radius/ulna fractures

Colles' fracture (1814)

Distal metaphyseal fracture within 2.5 cm of the articular surface; with dorsal displacement and angulation (silver fork deformity), with or without avulsion of ulnar styloid.

Three commonly used classifications:
1. Frykman's classification.
2. Universal classification.
3. Mayo classification.

Reference

Frykman G. Fracture of the distal radius including sequelae— shoulder–hand–finger syndrome, disturbance in the distal radioulnar joint and impairment of nerve function: a clinical and experimental study. *Acta Orthop Scand* **108** (Suppl): 1–153, 196.

Frykman's classification

Distal radial fracture	Distal ulnar fracture	
	Absent	Present
Extra-articular	I	II
Intra-articular involving radiocarpal joint	III	IV
Intra-articular involving distal radioulnar joint	V	VI
Intra-articular involving both radiocarpal and distal radioulnar joints	VII	VIII

Radius and

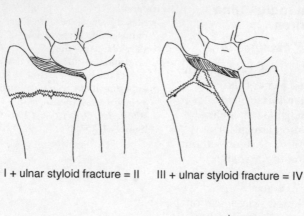

I + ulnar styloid fracture = II   III + ulnar styloid fracture = IV

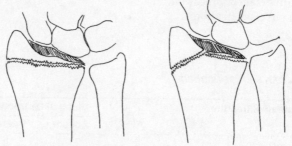

V + ulnar styloid fracture = VI   VII + ulnar styloid fracture = VIII

Fig. 45 Frykman's classification

Universal classification (modified from Gartland, Werley, Sarmiento)

Type I
Extra-articular; undisplaced.

Type II
Extra-articular; displaced.

Type III
Intra-articular; undisplaced.

Type IV
Intra-articular; displaced:
- A: reducible; stable.
- B: reducible; unstable.
- C: irreducible; unstable.

References

Gartland JJ Jr, Werley CW. Evaluation of healed Colles' fractures. *J Bone Joint Surg* 1951; **33A:** 895–907.

Sarmiento A, Pratt GW, Berry NC, Sinclair WF. Functional bracing in supination. *J Bone Joint Surg* 1975; **57A:** 311–317.

Radius and ulna

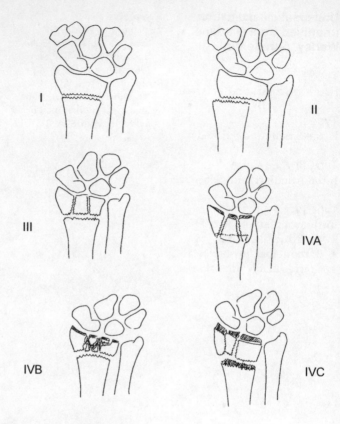

Fig. 46 Universal classification

Mayo classification (for intra-articular fracture of distal radius)

Type I
Undisplaced; intra-articular.

Type II
Displaced; involving radioscaphoid joint.

Type III
Displaced; involving radiolunate joint.

Type IV
Displaced; involving both radioscaphoid and radiolunate joints and the sigmoid fossa of the distal radius.

Reference
Rockwood CA, Green DP.
  Rockwood and Green's Fractures in Adults, 3rd edition.
  Philadelphia: JB Lippincott, 1991, p 589.

Radius an...

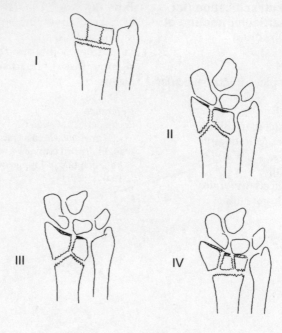

Fig. 47 Mayo classification

Smith's fracture (1854)

Reverse Colles' fracture: This is a volar angulated fracture of distal radius with garden spade deformity.

Modified Thomas' classification

Type I
Extra-articular.

Type II
Fracture line crosses into the dorsal articular surface.

Type III
Fracture line enters radiocarpal joint (volar Barton's fracture).

Reference
Thomas FB. Reduction of Smith's fracture. *J Bone Joint Surg* 1957; **39B:** 463–470.

Barton's fracture (1838)

This is a fracture dislocation or subluxation of distal radial rim, which is displaced dorsally or volarly with the hand and carpus. There are two main types:
- Volar Barton's fracture (Smith's type III).
- Dorsal Barton's fracture (intra-articular Colles' fracture).

Reference
Barton JR. Views and treatment of an important injury to the wrist. *Med Exam* 1838; **1:** 365.

Chauffeur's fracture (back-fired fracture)

This is a fracture of the radial styloid.

Radius and ulna

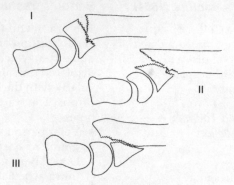

Fig. 48 Modified Thomas' classification

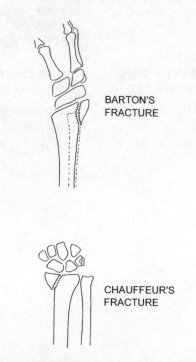

BARTON'S
FRACTURE

CHAUFFEUR'S
FRACTURE

Fig. 49 Barton's and Chauffeur's fractures

Carpus

Scaphoid fractures

Herbert's classification

Type A
Acute fractures; stable.
- A1: tubercle fracture.
- A2: waist fracture, incomplete.

Type B
Acute fracture; unstable.
- B1: waist fracture, complete.
- B2: transverse waist fracture, complete.
- B3: proximal pole fracture.
- B4: trans-scaphoid perlunate dislocation of the carpus.

Type C
Delayed union; widening of fracture line, development of cysts adjacent to the fracture line.

Type D
Established non-union.
- D1: fibrous non-union.
- D2: pseudarthrosis.

Reference
Herbert TJ. Scaphoid fractures and carpal instability. *Proc R Soc Med* 1974; **67:** 1080.

Carpus

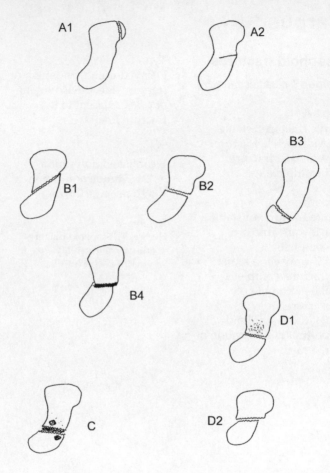

Fig. 50 Herbert's classification

Lunate fractures

Fractures of lunate are uncommon, and often missed; at least until they progress to osteochondrosis of the lunate at which they become symptomatic (Kienbock's disease).

Lichtman and Stahl classification (radiographic stages of Kienbock's disease)

Stage I
Linear or compression fracture.

Stage II
Sclerosis, collapse of radial border.

Stage III
Fragmentation, collapse, loss of height, capitate proximal migration.

Stage IV
Advanced collapse, cystic changes, scaphoid rotation, osteophyte of the radiocarpal joint.

References

Lichtman DM, Alexander AH, Mack GR, Gunter SR. Kienbock's disease: update on silicone replacement arthroplasty. *J Hand Surg* 1982; **7A**: 343.

Stahl F. On lunatomalacia (Kienbock's disease): a clinical and roentgenological study, especially on its pathogenesis and the late results of immobilization treatment. *Acta Chir Scand* 1947; **45** (Suppl 126): 1–33.

Carpus

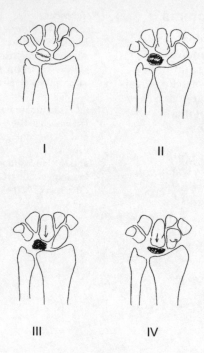

Fig. 51 Lichtman–Stahl classification

Hand

Thumb metacarpal (base) fractures

Type I: Bennet's fracture (1882)

Intra-articular fracture dislocation of the base of the thumb with a volar lip fragment from the metacarpal shaft. The shaft is displaced radially and dorsally at the base by the adductor pollicis longus. The pull of the adductor pollicis on the distal shaft increases the displacement of the base in abduction.

Type II: Rolando's fracture (1910)

Intra-articular fracture which in addition to the volar lip fragment of Bennet's fracture dislocation has a large dorsal fragment resulting in a Y or T shaped intra-articular fracture.

Type III: extra-articular fracture
- III A: transverse fracture line.
- III B: oblique fracture line.

Type IV: epiphyseal fracture

References

Bennet EH. Fractures of the metacarpal bones. *Dublin J Med Sci* 1882; **73:** 72–75.

Green DP, O'Brien E. Fractures of the thumb metacarpal. *South Med J* 1972; **65:** 807.

Rolando S. Fracture de la base du premier métacarpien: et principalement sur une variété non encore décrite. *Presse Med* 1910; **18:** 303–304.

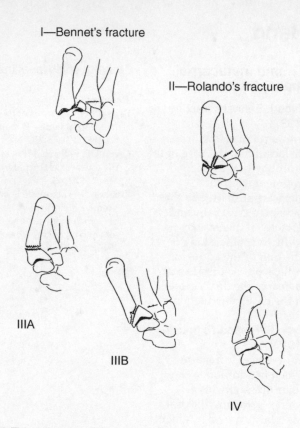

I—Bennet's fracture

II—Rolando's fracture

IIIA

IIIB

IV

Fig. 52 Thumb fracture: I, Bennet's; II, Rolando's; III, extra-articular; IV, epiphyseal

Distal phalangeal fractures

Extra-articular: Kaplan's classification
- Longitudinal.
- Transverse.
- Comminuted.

Reference
Kaplan L. The treatment of fractures and dislocations of the hand and fingers. Technique of unpadded casts for carpal, metacarpal and phalangeal fractures. *Surg Clin North Am* 1940; **20:** 1695–1720.

Intra-articular: mallet fracture (fracture of the dorsal articular surface of the distal phalanx—usually one-third or greater)

Wehbe and Schneider classification

Type I
Bony injury of varying extent without subluxation of the joint.

Type II
Fractures associated with joint subluxation.

Type III
Epiphyseal and physeal injuries.
   Each type is further subdivided into three types:
- A: fracture fragment less than one-third of the articular surface.
- B: fracture from one-third to two-thirds of the articular surface.
- C: fracture of more than two-thirds of the articular surface.

Reference
Wehbe MA, Schneider L. Mallet fractures. *J Bone Joint Surg* 1984; **66A:** 658–669.

Hand

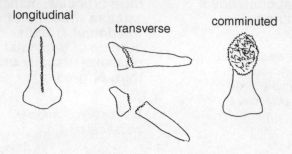

Fig. 53 Kaplan's classification

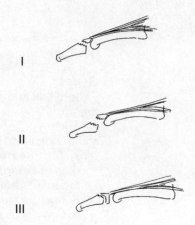

Fig. 54 Wehbe–Schneider classification